Renew Your Memory

Obtain an Unlimited Powerful Memory

Disclaimer

The author and publisher of this eBook have used their best efforts in preparing it. The author and publisher make no representation or warranties with respect to the accuracy, applicability, or completeness of the contents of this resource.

The information contained in this eBook is strictly for educational purposes. Therefore, if you wish to apply the ideas contained herein, you are taking full responsibility for your actions.

Trademarks mentioned in this book are property of their respective owners and may not be used without written permission. The fact that organizations, or websites are referred to in this work as examples does not mean that the author endorses the information, the company or website.

Readers should be aware that the information listed in this work may have changed or disappeared between when this book was written and when it is read.

Table of Contents

Introduction

This eBook will not only help in increasing and renewing a person's memory, but will also assist in reaching the peak of having a powerful memory. This is a guide for a greater understanding of what memories are made of, how well do we really remember things and how are all these are connected to the one almighty brain. It will unravel all the secrets of the human mind and how the memory can help in recalling things, events and learning experiences that had occurred or occurring in life.

All questions regarding achieving a powerful memory will be answered in this eBook. Why does the brain forget? How do I remember things quickly? What are the things that I can do to not easily forget? Can I achieve optimum brain power? How do people memorize the order of a standard deck of card or memorize a lengthy speech? How is that even possible? All these will be answered thoroughly in a simple and direct manner.

There will be various exercises, memory training and practical tests included in this eBook. This will also include visual and sound associations, techniques, and tips on how to achieve optimum memory. All these things will be discussed in these chapters. Meditation techniques to help increase memory will also be presented in this eBook, such as the memory palace technique and the loci method, how it is performed and where it is derived.

This book will help in understanding the unlimited capabilities of the brain and how it can be achieved. This will defy the mind to enhance its connections with brain cells and the memory. The brain needs to be regularly challenged in order to attain its uttermost performance.

Chapter 1:
Memory, a brief history and why we can actually increase and learn forever

Why do humans remember just about everything? The human brain can remember events, skills, habits, and experiences. The sum of what is remembered is called a memory. The word "memory" originated form the Latin *memorormemoria* which means "remembering" or "mindful." Human memories are rich and can be amusing most of the time. These are formed by associating what we experience, such as events or happenings in which the brain associates all the senses to the things that are being experienced. These learning experiences are retained by the brain for a period. Even the single most memory of any happening in a human's life can be retrieved when stimuli are present during the time that it happened.

Although the brain is a powerful tool in remembering details, it is still far from perfect and the human memory is not considered as accurately reliable in terms of specific and actual details. Memories can be distorted or changed over time. One memory can be associated wrongly with another memory especially with a lot of factors and activities that had already occurred in a person's life. Others would write a diary or journal to help retain their memories exactly. It is hard to rely on memory alone when the brain is not properly trained in retaining information. It is better to take note and keep it for future references.

The brain has the ability to remember things with no limitations. But why is it that the brain is not capable of remembering all the detailed and exact information that had occurred? Retaining all these facts and specific details should be assessed in terms of speed and not in terms of its storage capacity. The system in the brain cannot write down all the information that is being experienced at the moment and these usually come faster.

Although not all humans can recall or remember facts, there are some that can retain too much amount of details and information. Studies show that retaining memories can be learned through series of exercises, cerebral trainings, and practical tests. This will require a lot of focus and concentration until the brains get used to it. If a person repetitively recalls and remembers a thing or a lesson learned, chances are the brain will retain the information. Constant practice and doing mind exercises have proved to be beneficial in recalling memories and storing information.

Increasing learning through memory

Can humans ever have unlimited memory? Can remembering increase learning abilities? Memories are called the mental records that are retained in the human brain. The stored information is an access to the past, habits, skills, and everything that has happened in a person's life. The three stages of a memory process constitute encoding, data storage and information retrieval. The encoding phase sends the information to the brain and is filed into the most substantial compartment. The brain cells then process the stimuli and the information is translated. During the storage stage, the brain must retain these encoded

data for a longer time. Information retrieval is basically just retrieving the data out of the brain which translates into what the senses are getting signals from the brain.
It is hard to imagine memory without learning.

Learning new things means adding more information to the brain. However, memory may be a factor in which what is learned may be diminished over time. Sometimes the brain can be a bit loose with the presence of external factors such as lack of focus, lack of understanding, unstable emotions, depression or not paying too much attention to details. If the brain is processing more than one data in a class lesson, and the student is distracted or not paying attention, most likely the data will not be retained by the learner.

Memory indeed increases learning. The new experiences in a person's life such as learning new language or learning a new skill are associated with having a good and focused memory. If a person is learning the French language, it will signal the brain that something new is being processed by the mind or if the person is learning to play a piano for the first time. This will trigger the brain to focus and give additional effort to digest what's being learned or spoken.

Remember, listening or reading during class does not necessarily mean a student is actually learning. Learning is better achieved not just by doing but most importantly by reflecting on what was done. A student can better understand or learn a science project by doing experiments rather than just by listening to the teacher or reading books and study materials. Reflecting and analyzing leads to better learning as compared to just merely listening to lectures or reading books without really understanding its content. The social-emotional part of the memory can also make any learning experience unforgettable. Memory enhancing activities such as cooperative learning is encouraged in classes or even in other group activities outside school. This type of learning can also be practice in the office or any group activities.

Chapter 2:
How Does the Memory Work and Why Do Humans Forget?

How exactly does the brain retain information? How do memories work? It is believed that memory is similar to a cabinet full of files but the mechanisms are far more dynamic than that of the filing cabinet theory. The ability to retain a memory greatly depends on how the experiences and events are being translated in the brain.

The nerve cells in the brain communicate from neuron to neuron systems. It is basically neurons talking to each other with the presence of chemical signals inside the brain. It is the strength coming from the neuron connections that determines how these memories are made. If the strength is properly sustained, then it is where a memory is finally formed.

It is the brain that consciously registers any memory that has occurred and is automatically encoded, then the brain gathers and consolidates the information. This is when the brain signals for retrieval of information whenever it is needed.

The brain can easily configure itself and it is also a muscle. Since the brain is an organ, it is also susceptible to wearing, tearing, and being damaged as a person ages. When the brain is not used, it will lead to its possible memory deterioration.

Long-term and short-term memory

How long are memories stored in the brain? When the brain is storing memory, it is actually storing information. What determines what type of memory is being stored depends on the length of how it is stored in the brain. Both types of memories' capacity to store weakens as a person ages and other conditions that may have an adverse effect on the memory.

The first type of memory is known as the long-term memory. This is a system in the brain where all the information are stored, managed or used for retrieving information. Long term memory is further classified into several categories.

The second type is the short-term memory or sometimes called the working memory. As the term short denotes that information is only stored for a short time in the mind before it is transferred to the long-term memory or being terminated.

Why do people forget?

What's the reason behind why people forget things? A lot of reasons were proposed on how and why memories deplete or decrease in capacity over time.

People may tend to forget due to failure in storing information. When a person loses an information, the main reason for this is that the information gathered never really reaches the long-term memory. One example is when a person tries to picture out a fast food chain logo then tries to compare it with the actual logo. Mostly the color is easier to remember but the smaller details are forgotten. That is how the brain works.

There is also a theory known as the interference theory wherein the existing or current memories interfere with another memory that's already been stored. This happens when a memory recalled has similarities with the stored information in the brain. This is where interference is most likely to happen. One basic example is when a person attends a birthday party of the same exact person every year. Chances are the minor details will be forgotten and only obvious details such as drinking and eating will be remembered but the kind of drinks or types of food served is hardly recalled. In a proactive interference, the old memories usually never let the new memory remembers while in a retroactive interference, it happens when a new information restricts the brains capacity to recall a past information.

There are also moments in life wherein a person, no matter how hard they try, the memories are never recalled. This is called the decay theory. When an information stored is not rehearsed or retrieved for a long time it will have high chances of diminishing. Tracing a memory becomes harder and important details begin to disappear from the thoughts. This is probably the most common reason why a person forgets things or probably never remembers them.

Remembering is an important way of empowering the memory. It makes people think, decide, analyze situations, react to circumstances, able to learn new knowledge and imagine things. Forgetting some life details is not really a bad thing. Just imagine if all the things that had happened in life are remembered even the smallest details of every instances of every second in a person's life, that would be too much for the brain to handle and process.

Chapter 3:
Meditation Technique to Increase Memory

It is no surprise that meditation and memory are closely interconnected with each other. Meditation, in a good way can attribute remarkable structural changes to the brain. It can enhance the memory and improve a person's attention to details and regain focus. Meditation aims to give peace of mind and calmness to everyone.

Mindfulness Medication Technique

This is one of the most popular techniques in meditation. This technique requires focused attention. If a person is performing multi-tasking errands like chatting, answering phones, updating sheets and encoding data, it should be a lot more stressful than just doing a single job. However, studies show that if a person practices this kind of meditation technique, the multiple tasks become manageable and enables that person to stay sharp and focused even with numerous tasks assigned. This technique clears and refreshes the mind. Here are some known benefits of mindfulness meditation:

It can help a person remember a subconscious memory. Meditation allows the brain to be free from worry or unwanted thoughts that can create distraction. This process allows the brain to tap other memories and enables a person to remember an event or thing that may have already been forgotten. This is the time when the brain is clear and can have access to these hidden memories stored in the brain.

It strengthens the mind. Using the mind as the core of this technique enables the brain to achieve high levels of concentration and better focus. Through this technique, the mental muscles function and lessens the chances of experiencing early signs of memory loss and mental fatigue.

Meditation may help slow down the ageing process. When a person is in a lot of stress, the brain loses its focus, alertness and sharpness and most of the time makes memories deteriorate as a person ages. Meditation can somehow aid to the relaxation of the brain and makes a person become calmer thus minimizing the worries and could slow down ageing.

Breathing Meditation Technique (Belly Breathing)

This is one of the preferred breathing techniques because it's effective, simple and can easily be followed by anyone. It uses the diaphragm to find proper breathing muscle control. It can also be done anywhere as it relaxes, calms the mind and eases anxiety fast. If a person feels uneasy or restless, doing the belly breathing can definitely lessen the unwanted feeling. This simple breathing technique can be easily learned and followed. Belly breathing is better practiced sitting on a chair.

1. Find a comfortable place and take a seat. Sit up straight.
2. Align the head and the chin properly and keep it straight.
3. Just relax the body.
4. Place one hand above the chest while the other hand is placed just below the navel.

5. Inhale through the nose and exhale slowly and fully through the nose.

6. The breathing must go deeper into the lungs and moving lower to the body.

7. The upper body and the ribs are not needed for this breathing technique, relax these muscles.

8. Repeat exercise until the stomach is expanding more than the ribs and chest. This technique relaxes the upper torso and supplies the body with oxygen.

Cycling Sense Meditation Technique

This meditation technique requires a person to sit on a comfortable place and relax the muscles of the body. This technique is highly dependent on concentration and can be done between ten to thirty minutes. In order to reach the peak of awareness there will be cycling patterns through the senses. This enables a person to focus, concentrate and be fully immersed in whatever is being focused on. Focusing enables a person to improve memories.

First is to focus on vision. Scan the room using the eyes and focus on the sight, the different colors and even the textures of every object in the surrounding. Notice everything around by using the sense of sight. Just observe and don't mind yourself for a moment. Focus on the sight only and everything it sees around.

Next thing is to focus on hearing. Notice the breathing patterns of your body. Concentrate on the sound of the wind, sounds on the streets, sounds of people around and other sounds that can be heard. Again, just focus on the hearing and nothing else.

Now be aware using the sense of taste and smell. Take a look around the room and find something edible or anything that might be fragrant or anything that has a smell. If there is something to eat in the room go ahead and grab one. Smell it and enjoy its aroma. Get lost with the aroma and finally taste it and enjoy every bite and just focus on the food inside the mouth. Again focus on the food and forget about yourself first.

Now it's time to focus on body awareness. Use the sense of touch to feel the clothing unto the skin. Imagine its softness or roughness on the body. Also notice the body for tensions. Relax the muscles in the body and make sure the body is in a good posture. Also feel your balance by slowly twisting the body into several positions. Find where the sense of balance is and release any body tension and sit comfortably.

Lastly, be aware of the sense of time. Think first of what the past held and what the future holds. Then keep your focus on the present situation until everything is focused on the present state.

These steps can be repeated once again after all the steps are done until the body is comfortable in doing the meditation technique. This is a good way of separating the body from the senses and lets a person focus more on one thing without being diverted.

Chapter 4:
Memory training, practice and ways to associate and remember

Even the top names in the memorizing world have normal brains too. What makes them different is the effort and time they have given into enhancing their memory from only being capable of remembering basic thoughts for a short period, to a longer time. This includes memorizing exceptional patterns and complex things that an average person finds hard to do.

Visual Associations

Why does a person continue to forget details of an image or an object even if it was repeatedly viewed over and over again? The visual association can make a person remember almost all the details if this trick is properly applied. There are three basic steps in visualization and association.

1. *Using substitute words*. Sometimes there are concepts that are hard to remember and visualize. The secret to this is to substitute by converting hard concepts, unusual words or symbols into portions, and think of any memorable object, event or name that can be easily associated with it. This is called creating mental connection and for most people visualization is the easiest way to do this.

2. *Creating mental images*. To obtain solid mental connection to a new learning or information it must be notable enough to be remembered. Can any of you remember what you wore two weeks ago? It is easier to remember significant details or events such as wedding day, the first airplane ride or first time visit to a foreign country. Same is true with creating mental images, it is pronounced and easily identifiable. The trick is to think of the object as bigger, to better picture the object in the mind. Also, try to think of the object a lot or make an action within the image.

3. *Associating images together*. This is now the step where the images are being associated together to come up with a less complex image that can easily be recalled by the brain. The image formed should be something familiar or have a personal connection to the person for better recall.

Song and Memory Association

Listening to music or hearing a particular song on the playlist can bring out memories. It has been studied scientifically that music and memory have an extraordinary relationship. Whenever a favorite song that is intimate to a person is being played, a burst of memories just suddenly appear upon hearing the beat and lyrics. Take for example, a graduation song was played over the radio and the person hearing it suddenly recalls all significant graduation memories that they could remember. There is an instant connection between music and memory in a person's life. It's like creating a personal identity through musical connection and association. Even persons with dementia have shown to be responsive to music and are able to recall specific events while listening.

Several scientific studies prove that music has massive effects on the emotions and cognitive system of a human. It instantly stirs and stimulates precise emotions and later controls the cognitive functions of the brain.

Memory Sports

This type of sport was developed in the early 90's. The contestants are given different forms of information which they will memorize such as memorizing order of cards in random order. The completion also has guidelines to follow. Memory sports gathers the best of the best memory champions in the world and together they compete for titles. This is a sport solely requiring mental power and it inspires a lot of kids and adults to try memory games, and it even becomes a hobby for some.

Other ways to remember

A person with a good memory is usually associated with being smart, knowledgeable and intelligent. But memorization and memory recall can be achieved through proper training and technique. Here are other ways to remember and recall things easily:

Use of mnemonics. This method is basically assigning a letter to words to form acronyms that can easily be remembered by the brain. The most common example of this is the ROYGBIV (**R**ed **O**range **Y**ellow **G**reen **B**lue **I**ndigo **V**iolet) which stands for the seven colors of the rainbow. Anyone could be creative in creating their own mnemonics. It's a matter of associations or it could be relating it to personal experiences.

Writing the things to be memorized. This is another strategy most students make use of in recalling lessons better. Writing down notes is more effective than just listening alone. This method teaches a person to retain information and lessons better. Others would write the same thing over and over again just to make sure everything is well-remembered. It's really up to people on what method best works for them.

Chunking larger data into smaller pieces. This method is usually helpful in remembering numbers. Take for example the numbers746908173, if it is chunked as "746", "908"and "173" it is much easier to recall than memorizing seven digits all at once. Chunking enables the brain to recall details in portions before connecting it as one large data. This method is best used when memorizing cellphone numbers.

Converting words into images. Humans remember images better than words. The more vivid the picture in the mind, the more it is likely to be remembered. A person is given the sentence: "Larry is riding a red motorcycle while it's raining." In order to recall the sentence, that scene is converted to an image. In the picture, the motorcycle has a man riding on it and in order to remember the name "Larry" he could engrave the name on the man's shirt. To have the rain effect Larry is being imagined as drenched while riding a motorcycle. This is where the whole picture is created in the brain and the sentence is easier to recall.

Chapter 5:
Stress and why it kills memory

Understanding two types of stress

Not all stress is considered deadly or toxic to a person. There are two known types of stress—the acute stress and another is the chronic stress. Facing an instant difficulty and getting over it would have the stress hormones of a person return to its normal state and not have a lasting effect, this is identified as acute stress. Depending on how the body reacts sometimes acute stress can be somewhat considered as good, as it helps peak a person's performance.

But if a person suffers from the long-lasting effects of stress, it is considered as chronic stress, and it could lead to more fatal situations. It can cause a person to suffer from basic sickness to a more serious illness such as cancer. Chronic stress changes the brain's functions and lessens its ability to function properly and affects the overall body system.

Chronic stress can kill the brain

According to neuroscientists, chronic stress can lead to changes in the structure of the brain and even affect its functions. Studies show that those who suffer from chronic stress are more susceptible to mental problems related to mood disorders or have difficulty in learning. If the brain malfunctions, then the memory will suffer and recalling would be hard to do.

The neurons in the brain are generated in the hippocampus of the brain. This is the part of the brain where the person's memories, emotions and learnings happen. If a person experiences stress, the production of these neurons would cease. Newly formed neurons can be damaged even with just a single stressful episode in a person's life. That is why, stress must be properly managed before enters its chronic state. Stress is inevitable but it's always how a person deals with it and reacts to any situation that determines its effects. Why let stress put a person down? Situations should be controlled by humans, not by stress.

Stress can make a person irritable

If a person gets too irritable and distracted, there are tendencies that they could become forgetful. This is one of the signs that makes it clear that stress has a disparaging effect on the brain. This could also lead to being anti-social, depressed and having a weakened memory eventually. Stress can limit the production of new cells and can lead to the volume loss of the *prefrontal cortex* of the brain. This section is highly connected with the cognitive and emotional areas of the brain.

How to avoid stress and regain memory strength?

Don't be scared. Although stress can pull out the best in a person's life, there are still methods on how to avoid it and live a relaxing and worry free-life. These tips can help deal with stress and enable one enjoy life to the fullest.

Meditate and breathe deeply

Meditation and deep breathing can help in managing a person's anxiety. According to researchers, when a person meditates daily or engages in deep breathing exercises, it could help alter the neural pathways of the brain. This alteration can help in making a person more resilient to stress. Meditation can aid in releasing all the distracting thoughts of the mind and it counters the unwanted effects of stress since it lowers blood pressure and slows down heart rate.

Never stop learning new things

This does not mean that a person has to study in school all his life. Although advanced education is well associated to better learning and mental functioning, it does not necessarily mean that everything that needs to be learned can be found only in school. There are lots of mental activities that can be practiced, such as puzzles, reading books, writing stories, or finding a new hobby or acquiring a skill. Do something new and challenging, and the brain will get excited with having something new to learn. Learning is a never-ending process, it is best done with willingness and passion. When a person stops learning, the brain weakens.

Take care of personal health

To have a healthy mind, one should also have a healthy body. By eating proper diets containing enough nutrients needed by the body such as choosing natural foods over processed foods with no or less nutrition, the body will become healthier. Drinking the right amount of water and getting enough sleep also contributes to better memory and recall. Regular exercise not only tones the body but also strengthens it. A healthy body overall is very much related to having a healthy brain.

Know personal strengths

Knowing one's personal strength enables them to assess where more or less effort is needed in any situation. Learning one's strengths can help boost confidence and reduces the chances of experiencing stress. In memorizing, one should know how to use memory tools, may it be in the mind or physically present such as memo pads, phone reminders or to-do lists. Humans can't remember everything but knowing what the strengths are can definitely play an important role in recalling and memorizing.

Chapter 6:
Practice memory method

Who doesn't want to have fun while learning, right? It was already discussed that practicing memory can be attained through associations and rehearsals. There are lots of methods in practicing memory, and putting them into practice really does the trick, really nothing beats practice and perseverance. Here are some of the widely-used memory methods:

The Journey Method

This method is known for its simplicity and fun nature—if you like mind adventures, this is a very effective technique in remembering. It has been practiced for centuries or could be even longer than that. It was said to have been used by early Romans as they used this method to visualize how the items in their rooms should be accurately placed. The main principle of this technique is to imagine being on a journey where the items that are to be remembered are placed along the way. This method is best used if a sequence or list needs to be recalled.

Try this: Imagine going to the market and buying lots of stuff. Things to buy would be:

lemon, cookies, dishwashing liquid, pork ribs, potatoes, apples

Imagine the start of the journey from the doorstep going to the supermarket where the items will be bought.

Example: (First two items are done to better understand the method)

1. First stop, front door of the house: imagine **lemons** are scattered all over the floor mat.
2. Second stop, the mailbox: imagine **cookies** are flowing out of the mailbox.
3. ____
4. ____
5. ____
6. ____

The items should be properly associated with the already recognizable things or landmarks that can be found during the trip to the supermarket. This method requires a person to be already familiarized with the route before trying this method.

The Peg Method

This method is one of the most convenient and useful techniques in remembering. It uses visual images to provide pegs in which the memories are associated or hanged. It also helps remember the numerical sequence of all the items. Either the phonetic peg or rhyming peg can be used in learning this method.

Rhyming Peg

This method has been found useful in memorizing short lists. This can be effective with as much as 20 items and by using words that rhyme to form the pegs. By doing this method a person could significantly improve their memory skill.

Try this: Memorize the items below and see how well you scored. In the next column try supplying, using own words and continue memorizing combining both columns. In item number one—the number 'one' rhymes with 'sun'. Same is true with the succeeding numbers.

1. Sun	11. ______________
2. Crew	12. ______________
3. Sea	13. ______________
4. Floor	14. ______________
5. Chives	15. ______________
6. Bricks	16. ______________
7. Heaven	17. ______________
8. Bait	18. ______________
9. Sign	19. ______________
10. Den	20. ______________

Continue and practice without looking at the list until recollection of the items has greatly improved. For a more challenging test, try creating an image that comes with the list or to complicate things, add details such as color, shape, texture or feelings in the description to level up memory skills.

The Celebrity Method

For those who are fond of celebrities or enjoys watching movies and TV shows this method will definitely work. Almost everybody watches movies so this might be applicable to almost everyone. This method is not limited only to Hollywood celebrities, it could also include politicians, fantasy or cartoon characters, historical figures and just about any famous person. This method makes use of picturing celebrities as part of the scene and relates the information with them.

To be able to remember something, associate that thing with a famous celebrity or figure. This will make remembering more exciting and fun. For example a person met someone with the name Elvis, picturing that person as a singer and holding a guitar makes it easier to recall the person's name rather than just hearing the name Elvis.

Try this:

- A guy from the club was wearing a red hood and kind of resembled Jay-Z. The girl next to her had a common face and the only prominent thing on her face was a mole on the right upper lip and her name was Reina. Imagine how you would remember their names by associating them with celebrities.

- During a geography lesson one of the maps was shaped like Mickey Mouse. Another was shaped like a tennis racket. One of the nations is governed by a President with a name that rhymes with Harry Potter. Create a scenario of how to associate this with the already known information.

Chapter 7:
Memory Palace Technique or also called the Method of Loci

This technique is based on the fact that humans are better at remembering places. The term "memory palace" is a comparison to any familiar place or location that a person can visualize and easily imagine. Memory palace is also known as journey method or the loci method. This method is known to be one the oldest techniques of mnemonic system. The word "loci" originated form the word locus meaning location. Loci is the plural term for this word in which it was derived. Although this method has several names, the technique being used is all the same. The technique enables a person to remember better by storing information in these familiar places. This will serve as a guide to recall and improve memory with constant brain training and practice.

Memory palace or loci method was practiced by the Greeks and Romans more than 2,000 years ago. This technique was widely used in the ancient times during speech delivery. Talking without notes appears to be far more impressive than those who have copies of their speech in front of them.

This is how it works:

1. *Choosing the palace.* In this step the person must choose a location that is very familiar along with its surroundings as well. Remember that this technique is only effective if the person has very good mental skill and can walk and roam around easily. The best place to start with is inside the house.

2. *Pay attention to details.* What's the first thing that can be seen in a house? For example while walking to the dining room, a sparkly large chandelier is hanging up above the ceiling or while walking in the bathroom there's a large silver mirror hanging above the sink. Remember and store these distinctive details inside the brain. This will later on serve as a storage bin for the information.

3. *Visualize the whole palace inside the head*. Memorize each room and each distinctive object, set, equipment or furniture in that room. Repeatedly visit each place mentally and memorize every route of the palace that is imagined inside the head. Make sure everything in that house is memorized and imprinted in the brain.

4. *Associate it with things to be remembered*. Once every route, rooms and paths are mastered begin now by associating these stored details to the things that needs to be remembered. For example, the image of the whole place is already inside the head then there is a need to memorize a list of the things to buy for the party. This is where association begins. Imagine the chandelier as a balloon floating over the ceiling or the countertop in the kitchen full of wine, this is how the memory is trained.

5. *Revisit the palace*. This time a person has already made a route in the house and has successfully associated the list to every part of the house. To better train the mind, it is suggested to revisit the

route again and master it by doing the mental walk. Keep on practicing until everything seems normal and the brain is not having a hard time recalling.

Try this:

- The team is planning a bridal shower for your coworker to be held at a bar few blocks away from the office. The things assigned to you were to buy the following: party balloons, stockings, cake, pillows, ribbons, party poppers. Now create a scenario by imagining the situation like it actually is happening. Use the loci method and apply the instructions above. Start from the front door of the office.

- In a chemistry class, the professor said that all the elements in a periodic table must be memorized. Use this technique to create and place storage bins in selected rooms or places at school or any familiar place. Imagine where all the noble gases must be stored, it could be in the library or canteen. Be imaginative and try to fill all the rooms with all the elements.

Chapter 8:
How to develop a photographic memory

Ever wonder how people can retain so much information in their brains and recall details exactly the way it is? Is this even possible? Having a photographic memory is a skill and can be learned. Anyone can have photographic memory as long as there is willingness to learn. The mind works best with images and not with repetitions that is why associating with pictures is more achievable than just repeating the words all over again. Visual imagination is the secret to attaining this. The basic step is to learn to memorize basic patterns and categorize items accordingly.

Improve Overall Memory

As the body needs nutrients to function, the memory also needs proper care and exercise to operate effectively. When a person takes care of the body, it affects the brain and all its functions including memory retention. The brain controls all the system functions in the body.

Getting enough sleep is one of the basic techniques to improve the overall being of the memory. The sleep process reboots the brain and enables us to process all the information captured and absorbed during that day. The brain consolidates all the data and stores them accordingly and in the right places. The significant details are retained while insignificant details are discarded.

Proper diet and regular exercise also helps in maintaining the health of the memory and the overall mental health. Exercise increases blood and oxygen circulation in the body which would mean more oxygen is being supplied to the brain. The right amount of water must also be consumed in a day for the body system to function effectively. Stress is unavoidable, that's why it is important to manage it well. Chronic stress can lead to many harmful and destructive health effects eventually. Smoking, excessive caffeine and alcohol must be taken in moderate amounts or be avoided. It is a matter of choosing a healthy lifestyle and living a happy life.

Also, try to practice visualizing what the plans for the day would be. Visualize how it would happen. If possible, make plans B and C during visualization just in case the original plan does not work. This way there is anticipation going on and pre-planning is done so when the task is present it becomes easier to maneuver. These things can help improve overall memory, can help in developing photographic memory and thought awareness. This creates a healthy atmosphere for significant memory growth and cognitive enrichment.

Using the Military Method

Why is it even called the military method? This method has been used by the military for almost seven decades and has been said to be effective. This is also where it derived the "military" in its name. This method can be done for a minimum of 15 minutes per day in a span of a month or so. See below steps for instructions.

1. Go find a dark room and must be free from any distraction.
2. Find a lamp or anything bright that can be used as light.
3. Try to find a position near the light for easier access when turning on the light.

4. Now get a paper and cut a hole with a rectangular shape. About 1/4 of a standard book size.

5. Open a book and cover it with the paper with a hole and expose only a single paragraph of the book.

6. Start turning off the lights so the eyes can adjust to darkness.

7. Then, turn on the light and immediately turn it off in a matter of seconds. A visual imprint of the material will be created.

8. Slowly as the imprint fades, begin to flip the light on while the eyes are staring at the book.

9. Do this process over and over until all the words in the paragraph are in its proper order.

To know if the method is correctly followed, the paragraph must be imprinted in the mind and the person is able to read it inside the mind. Try the other paragraphs also and imprint as many images in the brain. This is how powerful a memory can work only if the right technique and training is used and practiced.

Chapter 9:
More brain power—Meditation, vitamins/minerals, fasting and autophagy

Brain power. The brain contains all the information that a person has, including experiences. It stores all the learnings and knowledge accumulated from the time a person started to learn and evaluate thoughts. Although the brain is a powerful tool of the past, it does not limit it to interpret present conditions or predict the future.

Meditation. It is known that meditation has beneficial effects on the body and mind. There are plenty of books, writings and information that discuss meditation and how it should be done. There is no such thing as the best meditation technique it really depends on where the person is comfortable and what works best.

There are two general types of meditation:

The *focused attention* which is a type of meditation that focuses only on a single object during the whole session. The object may be: a visualization, a mantra, a physical object, any body part or could be breathing patterns and a lot more. As soon as the person starts to get used to this kind of meditation, the attention and focus lengthens and lesser time for distraction have been developed. Popular examples of this are the Buddhist and Chakra meditations.

The second type is the *monitoring meditation,* which contrary to the focused attention, focuses on all possible aspects of a learning or an experience. This meditation however does not require judgment and attachment. It is a kind of non-reactive monitoring of any event. Some of the popular types of this meditation technique are Taoist meditation and *Vispassana* meditation.

Vitamins and Minerals. Eating food alone does not guarantee compete nutrient absorption from the body. Sometimes the food intake is not enough to supply the vitamins and minerals the body needs. In order to fill in those deficiencies, there are available daily supplementary multivitamins that can be taken. Although a lot of these supplements are present in the market, these nutrients can still be taken from organic green leafy vegetables and organic fruits. Since these are sometimes hard to grow or even find in the supermarket, this is where multivitamins come in handy and are useful.

The mind needs nourishment to have a well-balanced mental health and good memory.
But can a tablet really help enhance memory? According to scientists, vitamin B_{12} when taken together with Omega-3 could slow down the cognitive decline on patients with Alzheimer's disease. B_{12} can be taken as a supplement or it can be found naturally in poultry and fish products.

Folic acid is another vitamin B supplement that is good for the brain. It is mostly taken by pregnant women for better brain development of babies. It also improves alertness and boost memory of a person.

Magnesium is said to have protective powers against neurotoxins that harm the brain. This is also why patients that undergo brain surgery have to take magnesium first.

Fasting and autophagy

Fasting is such a common word and greatly understood by almost anyone. But what is autophagy and how does it work? Autophagy was derived from the Greek word *auto* meaning self and *phagein* meaning to eat. Literally the word means 'eating its own self.' This process is a kind of mechanism inside the body where it liberates or throws out the old cells that are no longer in use and replaces them with new cells.

But what is really the relationship between fasting and autophagy? Depriving the body from the nutrients it needs activates autophagy in the body. Fasting raises glucagon in the body and this boosts the process of autophagy. See now the relationship of the two? Fasting is very essential in autophagy which enables cellular cleansing, getting rid of the old cells and producing new ones.

Eating turns off the process of autophagy. This is when the body is high in glucose, protein and experiences decrease in glucagon level. This process can only be achieved through fasting or sometimes like others like to call it, dieting. The key here is balance. Excessive autophagy or too little can actually make a person sick.

Fasting and autophagy helps in boosting brain power. According to researchers, during fasting, the brain acts as if there is a stress happening to the system. The brain becomes more active when it is stressed. So when the body is hungry the brain seeks and craves for more food. During fasting no eating activity must be done three hours before going to sleep. This is just to contain a person's eating habit within the 8 hour gap period. After few weeks the body can adjust and adapt without feeling hungry even for more than 15 hours.

Chapter 10:
Practice memory method: More advanced – the Alphabet system

The Alphabet System

This technique uses the peg memory but is more refined than the number system. It is most often used to remember plenty of items that are placed in a specific order. This way there will be no missing item on the list.

But first be familiarized with the phonetic alphabets.

A-C	F-J	K-O	P-T	U-Z
Alpha	Foxtrot	Kilo	Papa	Uniform
Bravo	Golf	Lima	Quebec	Victor
Charlie	Hotel	Mike	Romeo	Whiskey
Delta	India	November	Sierra	X-ray
Echo	Juliet	Oscar	Tango	Yankee
				Zulu

Phonetic alphabet can be very useful in substituting data with their equivalents. If a person wants to remember a password or lock code with 4 letters, J-W-V-C. Imagine Juliet is drinking Whiskey with Victor and Charlie.

Alternatively the letter A-Z can also be used as peg system. The alphabets are associated with something that needs to be remembered. This enables a person to remember up to 26 items since the alphabet system has 26 letters.

Try this:

Make a peg similar to this.

A= ape

B = bat

C = crab

Then associate them with the list of things that are needed to be bought in the grocery store: cheese, asparagus and tofu. Now connect everything and form an image out of the list.

- Picture the ape devouring on the cheese
- Picture the bat nibbling the asparagus
- Picture the crab with tofu on its claws

Upon arriving to the grocery store, recall using the alphabet pegs and start with the shopping. Assign your own pegs for each letter. It should be something easily remembered and of significance. Aside from using animals, people's names, food, objects, shapes, even sounds can also be associated to create alphabet pegs.

Try this:

Try to memorize this alphabet sequence. The sequence can be portioned if preferred. Depending on what technique is used.

D – H- B– D- S – G - S

Done? Now, these letters stand for the first letters of Snow White's seven dwarfs. D is for Doc, H is for Happy, D is for Dopey, S is for Sleepy, g is for Grumpy and S is for Sneezy. The sequence can be altered by putting all the D's and S's next to each other for better memory retention. Using this method, it is seen that to recall set of names just by remembering the first letter of their names is better.

- Try to make a sequence for the planets ranging from the smallest to the biggest and vice versa.

- Try also the alphabet system in memorizing all the presidents of America.

- For fast learners, try this method for all the continents and then all the countries that belong to each continent.

Isn't it fun? Creating personal techniques and strategies will really help improve the memory.

Conclusion

Now you know the fundamentals of improving memory. Hopefully, you have also learned various methods of boosting memory, mind training, and techniques to help manage mental health.

The book serves as a handy tool whenever you need to memorize or remember something important. The process is a lot easier and faster since everything that needs to be done and learned are contained in this eBook.

At the beginning of the eBook there were questions presented and by the end of the chapters those questions were answered in detail along with brain training exercises. There will be more exercises found at the end of this chapter. Feel free to try and do these mental exercises for the brain.

Always keep in mind the aim here is to achieve a powerful mind and develop a healthy memory. Do not just read but practice and apply. This eBook definitely helped in achieving those goals. Build a memory training program and the brain will thank you for that.

Those who participated in all of the brain training exercises find it easier to memorize and recall things. The exercises included here are practical and they can be applied to almost anything.

This is something worth learning and reading.

BONUS:
More brain training exercises

Brain training exercise #1

Try first this simple short term memory test. Look around you and find 15 objects and put them on top of the table. These items could be a ballpen, clip, sharpener, memo pad, bottle, spoon, etc. Try memorizing all the items for 10 seconds and then cover all the items with a cloth or large piece of paper. Recall as many as you can remember.

Brain training exercise #2

Read the list below and remember everything in order. There are 20 items on the list. Try to memorize and answer the next questions after that. No cheating. This test will test how photographic the memory can be.

1. Faded blue jeans

2. Pink plastic ribbon

3. Dusty round bowl

4. Broken bottle

5. Triangular box

6. Violet jacket

7. Crunchy cookie

8. Sweaty shirt

9. Messy table

10. Wooden chair

11. Ripped curtain

12. Glass window

13. Hair blower

14. Water jug

15. Red ball pen

16. Airplane

17. Pepper shaker

18. Motor bike

19. Green grass

20. Hot oven

Now cover the list with a paper or folder as long as the list is not showing. Now from just the memory alone, recall the following and write down on a piece of paper. The 4th item on the list, the 10th item, 16th and the 19th item. How many correct answers did you get? Was it challenging enough to memorize?

Brain training exercise #3

Memorize all the words in 5 minutes. Time can be extended for beginners and newbies. Write down all the words that you can remember on a piece of paper.

trip	beef	lass	Clue	Stone	three
grip	sweep	blast	Keen	Bone	bread
clap	stop	file	Oven	Cone	orange
vast	tart	drill	Shoe	Stork	block
tone	paint	grant	House	Phone	line
crown	stout	kiss	Bliss	Mouse	circle
bake	steak	stick	Bark	Crow	beak
spark	soap	clock	Brim	shine	bite
park	truck	kite	Soil	pine	coil

Did you get everything right? What method did you use? Was it effective? Keep on practicing using other sets of words or images.

Brain training exercise #4

Below are pictures of famous Hollywood directors with their name underneath the picture. Practice all the methods and techniques that were learned from this eBook and rate how many were recognized. If you want more challenging pictures you can try fictional characters or politicians from foreign countries.

1. Memorize their names alphabetically
2. Memorize names and describe their faces
3. Memorize in sequence

TIP: Associate the faces with someone familiar to you or maybe the name is similar with that of a person you personally know.

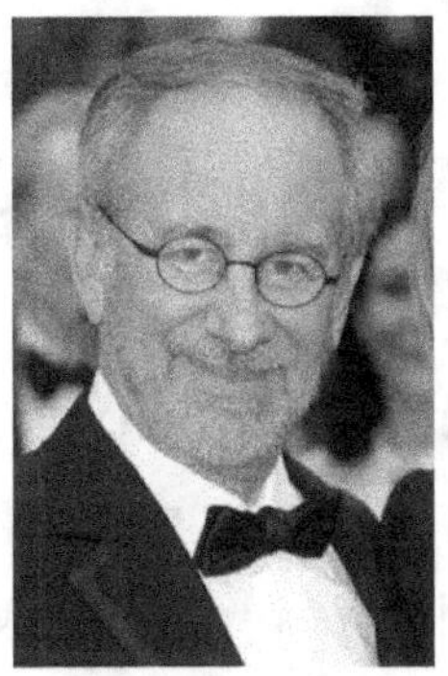

Image 1:
Steven Spielberg

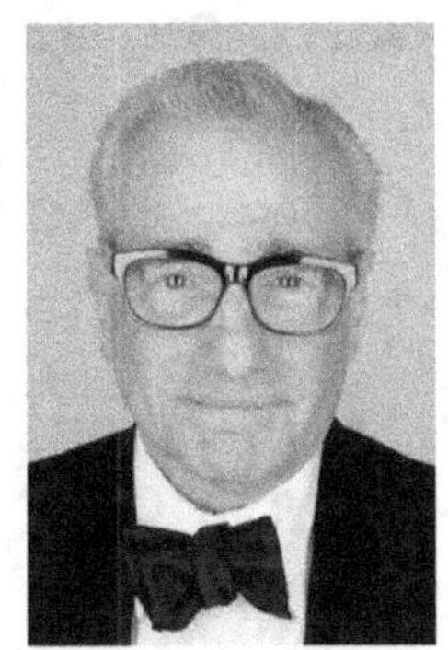

Image 2:
Martin Scorsese

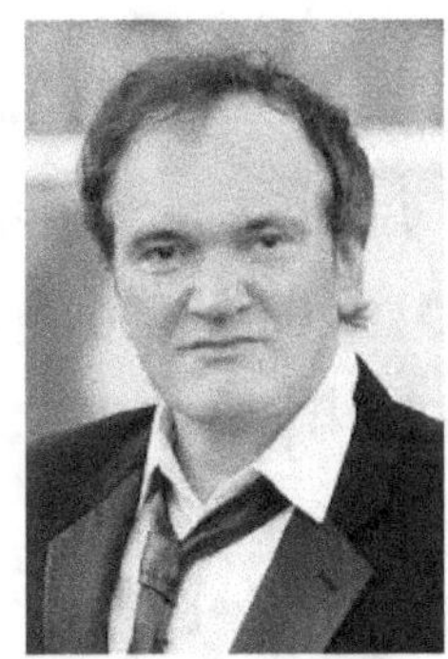

Image 3:
Quentin Tarantino

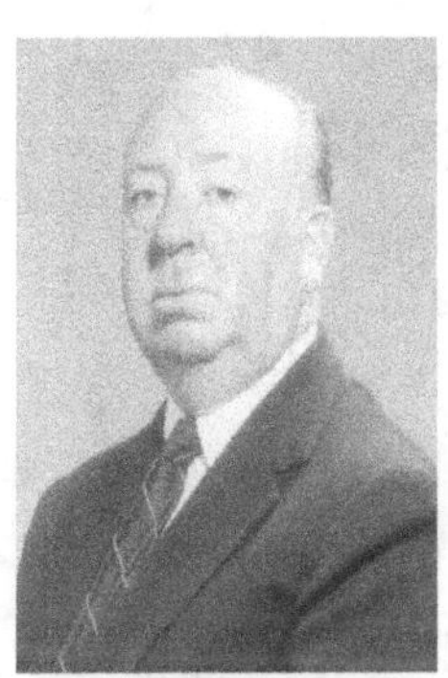

Image 4:
Alfred Hitchcock

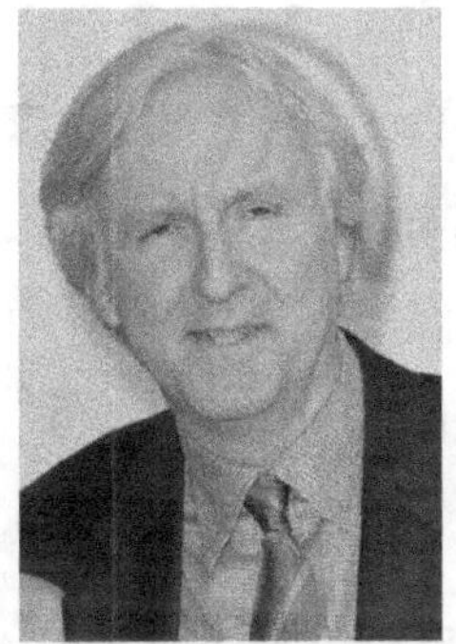

Image 5:
James Cameron

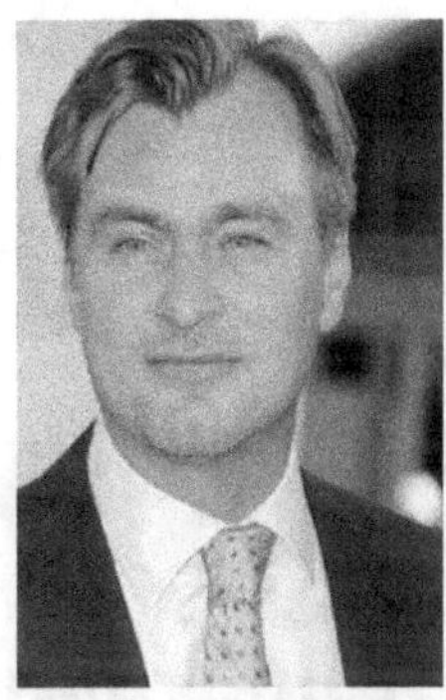

Image 6:
Christopher Nolan

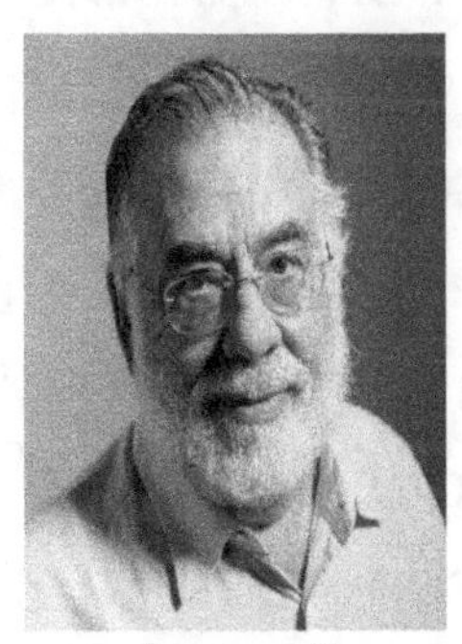

Image 7
: Francis Ford Coppola

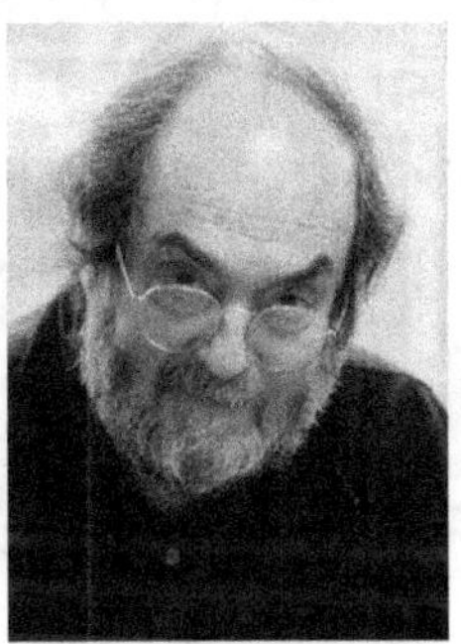

Image 10:
Stanley Kubrick

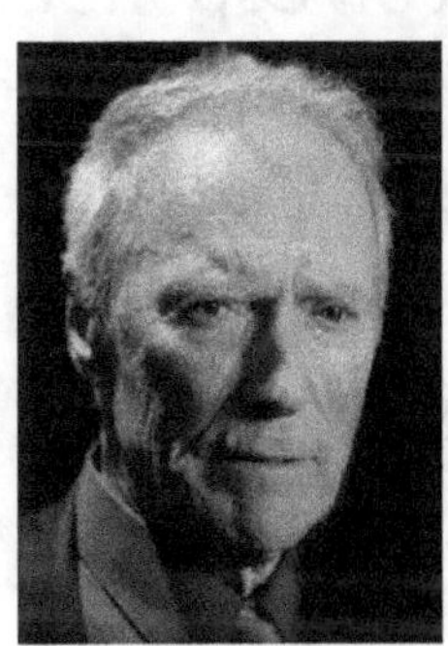

Image 9:
Clint Eastwood

Brain training exercise #5

Find a really interesting book of your preference. Choose something that you are really interested in. If you do not like books, try watching a new movie or find a newly released song and print the lyrics. Now, all you have to do, if you are reading a book or a movie, summarize it by writing it down on a piece of paper. If you are listening to a new song memorize its lyrics and sing along with the song to find out if the lyrics are memorized perfectly. These things must be done in the shortest possible time. Good luck and have fun learning!

Brain training exercise #6

Memorize the following countries and their corresponding capitals. These are some of the countries with hard to pronounce names. Ask someone to read out loud the country then guess the capital or you can do the other way around. If you want to be challenged, try recalling the list in alphabetical order or based on the current sequence. You can also try spelling out the words on a piece of paper.

You can do just about anything form this list. Apply all the techniques and methods learned from this eBook. Remmeber, no peeking! Enjoy the game!

Country	Capital
Moldova	Chisinau
Burundi	Bujumbura
Comoros	Moroni
Togo	Lomé
Liechtenstein	Vaduz
Vanuatu	Port Vila
Guinea-Bissau	Bissau
Saint Kitts and Nevis	Basseterre
Burkina Faso	Ouagadougou
Djibouti	Djibouti

Have fun memorizing!